Blood Pressure Logbook

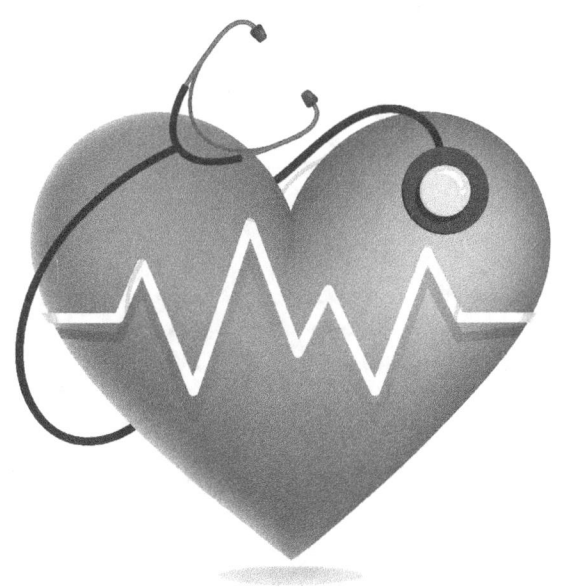

Doctor B. Telep

Copyright ©

All rights reserved. Doctor B. Telep
No parts of this publication may be reproduced, distributed, or transmitted in any form, or by any means, including photocopying, recording or other electronic or mechanical methods, without prior written permission from the publisher.

Reference Values

Blood Pressure	Systolic mm Hg (upper number)	Diastolic mm Hg (upper number)
Normal	Less than 120	Less than 80
Elevated	120 - 129	Less than 80
High blood pressure (hypertension stage I)	130 - 139	80 - 89
High blood pressure (hypertension stage II)	140 or higher	90 or higher
Hypertensive crisis (consult doctor immediately)	Higher than 180	Higher than 120

Date ....

Sleep quality and duration ....

Stress levels   1   2   3   4   5   6   7   8   9   10

Time	Systolic	Diastolic	Heart Rate

Exercise and daily activities   Water Intake ⬜⬜⬜⬜⬜⬜⬜

....
....
....
....
....
....
....
....
....
....
....
....
....
....
....
....

Breakfast	Lunch

Dinner	Snacks

Supplements	Medication

Date ....

Sleep quality and duration ....

Stress levels 1 2 3 4 5 6 7 8 9 10

Time	Systolic	Diastolic	Heart Rate

Exercise and daily activities   Water Intake ⬜⬜⬜⬜⬜⬜⬜

....

....

Breakfast	Lunch

....

....

....

....

....

Dinner	Snacks

....

....

....

....

Supplements	Medication

....

....

....

....

Date ....

Sleep quality and duration ....

Stress levels   1   2   3   4   5   6   7   8   9   10

Time	Systolic	Diastolic	Heart Rate

Exercise and daily activities   Water Intake ▯▯▯▯▯▯▯

....
....
....
....
....
....
....
....
....
....
....
....
....
....
....
....

Breakfast	Lunch
Dinner	Snacks
Supplements	Medication

Date ....

Sleep quality and duration ....

Stress levels   1   2   3   4   5   6   7   8   9   10

Time	Systolic	Diastolic	Heart Rate

Exercise and daily activities   Water Intake ⬜⬜⬜⬜⬜⬜⬜

....

....

....

Breakfast	Lunch

....

....

....

....

Dinner	Snacks

....

....

....

....

....

Supplements	Medication

....

....

....

....

Date ....

Sleep quality and duration ....

Stress levels   1   2   3   4   5   6   7   8   9   10

Time	Systolic	Diastolic	Heart Rate

Exercise and daily activities   Water Intake ☐☐☐☐☐☐☐

....
....
....
....
....
....
....
....
....
....
....
....
....
....
....
....

Breakfast	Lunch
Dinner	Snacks
Supplements	Medication

Date ....

Sleep quality and duration ....

Stress levels   1   2   3   4   5   6   7   8   9   10

Time	Systolic	Diastolic	Heart Rate

Exercise and daily activities   Water Intake ▢▢▢▢▢▢▢

....
....
....
....
....
....
....
....
....
....
....
....
....
....
....
....

Breakfast	Lunch

Dinner	Snacks

Supplements	Medication

Date ....

Sleep quality and duration ....

Stress levels   1   2   3   4   5   6   7   8   9   10

Time	Systolic	Diastolic	Heart Rate

Exercise and daily activities   Water Intake ▯▯▯▯▯▯▯

....

....

....

....

....

....

....

....

....

....

....

....

....

....

....

....

Breakfast	Lunch

Dinner	Snacks

Supplements	Medication

Date ....

Sleep quality and duration ....

Stress levels   1   2   3   4   5   6   7   8   9   10

Time	Systolic	Diastolic	Heart Rate

Exercise and daily activities   Water Intake ⬜⬜⬜⬜⬜⬜⬜

....
....
....
....
....
....
....
....
....
....
....
....
....
....
....
....

Breakfast	Lunch

Dinner	Snacks

Supplements	Medication

Date ....

Sleep quality and duration ....

Stress levels   1   2   3   4   5   6   7   8   9
10

Time	Systolic	Diastolic	Heart Rate

Exercise and daily activities   Water Intake ☐☐☐☐☐☐☐

....
....
....
....
....
....
....
....
....
....
....
....
....
....
....
....
....

Breakfast	Lunch

Dinner	Snacks

Supplements	Medication

Date ....

Sleep quality and duration ....

Stress levels   1   2   3   4   5   6   7   8   9   10

Time	Systolic	Diastolic	Heart Rate

Exercise and daily activities   Water Intake ☐☐☐☐☐☐☐

....
....
....
....
....
....
....
....
....
....
....
....
....
....
....
....

Breakfast	Lunch
Dinner	Snacks
Supplements	Medication

Date ....

Sleep quality and duration ....

Stress levels   1   2   3   4   5   6   7   8   9   10

Time	Systolic	Diastolic	Heart Rate

Exercise and daily activities   Water Intake ☐☐☐☐☐☐

....
....
....
....
....
....

Breakfast	Lunch

....
....
....
....
....

Dinner	Snacks

....
....
....
....
....

Supplements	Medication

Date ....

Sleep quality and duration ....

Stress levels   1   2   3   4   5   6   7   8   9   10

Time	Systolic	Diastolic	Heart Rate

Exercise and daily activities   Water Intake ⬜⬜⬜⬜⬜⬜⬜

....
....
....
....
....
....
....
....
....
....
....
....
....
....
....
....
....

Breakfast	Lunch

Dinner	Snacks

Supplements	Medication

Date ....

Sleep quality and duration ....

Stress levels 1 2 3 4 5 6 7 8 9 10

Time	Systolic	Diastolic	Heart Rate

Exercise and daily activities   Water Intake ☐☐☐☐☐☐☐

....
....
....
....
....
....
....
....
....
....
....
....
....
....
....

Breakfast	Lunch

Dinner	Snacks

Supplements	Medication

Date ....

Sleep quality and duration ....

Stress levels   1   2   3   4   5   6   7   8   9   10

Time	Systolic	Diastolic	Heart Rate

Exercise and daily activities   Water Intake ☐☐☐☐☐☐☐

....
....
....
....
....
....
....
....
....
....
....
....
....
....
....
....

Breakfast	Lunch

Dinner	Snacks

Supplements	Medication

Date ....

Sleep quality and duration ....

Stress levels   1   2   3   4   5   6   7   8   9
10

Time	Systolic	Diastolic	Heart Rate

Exercise and daily activities   Water Intake ☐☐☐☐☐☐☐

....
....
....
....
....
....
....
....
....
....
....
....
....
....
....
....

Breakfast	Lunch
Dinner	Snacks
Supplements	Medication

Date ....

Sleep quality and duration ....

Stress levels   1   2   3   4   5   6   7   8   9   10

Time	Systolic	Diastolic	Heart Rate

Exercise and daily activities   Water Intake ☐☐☐☐☐☐☐

....
....
....
....
....
....
....
....
....
....
....
....
....
....
....
....

Breakfast	Lunch
Dinner	Snacks
Supplements	Medication

Date ....

Sleep quality and duration ....

Stress levels   1   2   3   4   5   6   7   8   9 10

Time	Systolic	Diastolic	Heart Rate

Exercise and daily activities   Water Intake ☐☐☐☐☐☐☐

....
....
....
....
....
....
....
....
....
....
....
....
....
....
....
....
....

Breakfast	Lunch

Dinner	Snacks

Supplements	Medication

Date ....

Sleep quality and duration ....

Stress levels   1   2   3   4   5   6   7   8   9   10

Time	Systolic	Diastolic	Heart Rate

Exercise and daily activities   Water Intake ☐☐☐☐☐☐☐

....
....
....
....
....
....
....
....
....
....
....
....
....
....
....

Breakfast	Lunch

Dinner	Snacks

Supplements	Medication

Date ....

Sleep quality and duration ....

Stress levels   1   2   3   4   5   6   7   8   9   10

Time	Systolic	Diastolic	Heart Rate

Exercise and daily activities   Water Intake ☐☐☐☐☐☐☐

....
....
....
....
....
....
....
....
....
....
....
....
....
....
....

Breakfast	Lunch
Dinner	Snacks
Supplements	Medication

Date ....

Sleep quality and duration ....

Stress levels 1 2 3 4 5 6 7 8 9 10

Time	Systolic	Diastolic	Heart Rate

Exercise and daily activities   Water Intake ☐☐☐☐☐☐☐

....
....
....
....
....
....
....
....
....
....
....
....
....
....
....

Breakfast	Lunch

Dinner	Snacks

Supplements	Medication

Date ....

Sleep quality and duration ....

Stress levels   1   2   3   4   5   6   7   8   9   10

Time	Systolic	Diastolic	Heart Rate

Exercise and daily activities   Water Intake ▢▢▢▢▢▢▢

....
....
....
....
....
....
....
....
....
....
....
....
....
....
....
....

Breakfast	Lunch

Dinner	Snacks

Supplements	Medication

Date ....

Sleep quality and duration ....

Stress levels   1   2   3   4   5   6   7   8   9   10

Time	Systolic	Diastolic	Heart Rate

Exercise and daily activities   Water Intake ☐☐☐☐☐☐☐

....
....
....
....
....
....
....
....
....
....
....
....
....
....
....
....
....

Breakfast	Lunch

Dinner	Snacks

Supplements	Medication

Date ....

Sleep quality and duration ....

Stress levels   1   2   3   4   5   6   7   8   9   10

Time	Systolic	Diastolic	Heart Rate

Exercise and daily activities   Water Intake ▢▢▢▢▢▢▢

....
....
....
....
....
....

Breakfast	Lunch

....
....
....
....
....

Dinner	Snacks

....
....
....
....
....

Supplements	Medication

....

Date ....

Sleep quality and duration ....

Stress levels   1   2   3   4   5   6   7   8   9   10

Time	Systolic	Diastolic	Heart Rate

Exercise and daily activities   Water Intake ⬜⬜⬜⬜⬜⬜⬜

....
....
....
....
....
....
....
....
....
....
....
....
....
....
....
....

Breakfast	Lunch

Dinner	Snacks

Supplements	Medication

Date ....

Sleep quality and duration ....

Stress levels   1   2   3   4   5   6   7   8   9   10

Time	Systolic	Diastolic	Heart Rate

Exercise and daily activities   Water Intake ☐☐☐☐☐☐☐

....
....
....
....
....
....
....
....
....
....
....
....
....
....
....
....
....

Breakfast	Lunch

Dinner	Snacks

Supplements	Medication

Date ....

Sleep quality and duration ....

Stress levels   1   2   3   4   5   6   7   8   9   10

Time	Systolic	Diastolic	Heart Rate

Exercise and daily activities   Water Intake ☐☐☐☐☐☐☐

....
....
....
....
....
....
....
....
....
....
....
....
....
....
....
....

Breakfast	Lunch

Dinner	Snacks

Supplements	Medication

Date ....

Sleep quality and duration ....

Stress levels   1   2   3   4   5   6   7   8   9   10

Time	Systolic	Diastolic	Heart Rate

Exercise and daily activities   Water Intake ☐☐☐☐☐☐☐

....
....
....
....
....
....
....
....
....
....
....
....
....
....
....
....

Breakfast	Lunch

Dinner	Snacks

Supplements	Medication

Date ....

Sleep quality and duration ....

Stress levels   1   2   3   4   5   6   7   8   9   10

Time	Systolic	Diastolic	Heart Rate

Exercise and daily activities   Water Intake ☐☐☐☐☐☐☐

....
....
....
....
....
....
....
....
....
....
....
....
....
....
....
....

Breakfast	Lunch
Dinner	Snacks
Supplements	Medication

Date ....

Sleep quality and duration ....

Stress levels   1   2   3   4   5   6   7   8   9   10

Time	Systolic	Diastolic	Heart Rate

Exercise and daily activities   Water Intake ☐☐☐☐☐☐

....
....
....
....
....
....
....
....
....
....
....
....
....
....
....
....
....

Breakfast	Lunch

Dinner	Snacks

Supplements	Medication

Date ....

Sleep quality and duration ....

Stress levels   1   2   3   4   5   6   7   8   9   10

Time	Systolic	Diastolic	Heart Rate

Exercise and daily activities   Water Intake ⬜⬜⬜⬜⬜⬜⬜

....
....
....
....
....
....
....
....
....
....
....
....
....
....
....

Breakfast	Lunch

Dinner	Snacks

Supplements	Medication

Date ....

Sleep quality and duration ....

Stress levels   1   2   3   4   5   6   7   8   9   10

Time	Systolic	Diastolic	Heart Rate

Exercise and daily activities   Water Intake ▯▯▯▯▯▯▯

....
....
....
....
....
....
....
....
....
....
....
....
....
....
....
....

Breakfast	Lunch
Dinner	Snacks
Supplements	Medication

Date ....

Sleep quality and duration ....

Stress levels   1   2   3   4   5   6   7   8   9   10

Time	Systolic	Diastolic	Heart Rate

Exercise and daily activities   Water Intake ⬜⬜⬜⬜⬜⬜⬜

....

....

Breakfast	Lunch

....

....

....

....

....

Dinner	Snacks

....

....

....

....

Supplements	Medication

....

....

....

....

....

Date ....

Sleep quality and duration ....

Stress levels　　1　2　3　4　5　6　7　8　9 10

Time	Systolic	Diastolic	Heart Rate

Exercise and daily activities　　Water Intake ☐☐☐☐☐☐☐

....
....
....
....
....
....
....
....
....
....
....
....
....
....
....
....

Breakfast	Lunch

Dinner	Snacks

Supplements	Medication

Date ....

Sleep quality and duration ....

Stress levels   1   2   3   4   5   6   7   8   9   10

Time	Systolic	Diastolic	Heart Rate

Exercise and daily activities   Water Intake ⬜⬜⬜⬜⬜⬜⬜

....
....
....
....
....
....
....
....
....
....
....
....
....
....
....
....

Breakfast	Lunch

Dinner	Snacks

Supplements	Medication

Date ....

Sleep quality and duration ....

Stress levels   1   2   3   4   5   6   7   8   9   10

Time	Systolic	Diastolic	Heart Rate

Exercise and daily activities   Water Intake ☐☐☐☐☐☐☐

....
....
....
....
....
....
....
....
....
....
....
....
....
....
....

Breakfast	Lunch

Dinner	Snacks

Supplements	Medication

Date ....

Sleep quality and duration ....

Stress levels   1   2   3   4   5   6   7   8   9   10

Time	Systolic	Diastolic	Heart Rate

Exercise and daily activities   Water Intake ▯▯▯▯▯▯▯

....
....
....
....
....
....
....
....
....
....
....
....
....
....
....
....

Breakfast	Lunch

Dinner	Snacks

Supplements	Medication

Date ....

Sleep quality and duration ....

Stress levels   1   2   3   4   5   6   7   8   9   10

Time	Systolic	Diastolic	Heart Rate

Exercise and daily activities   Water Intake ☐☐☐☐☐☐☐

....

....

....

....

....

....

....

....

....

....

....

....

....

....

....

....

Breakfast	Lunch

Dinner	Snacks

Supplements	Medication

Date ....

Sleep quality and duration ....

Stress levels   1   2   3   4   5   6   7   8   9   10

Time	Systolic	Diastolic	Heart Rate

Exercise and daily activities   Water Intake ☐☐☐☐☐☐☐

....
....
....
....
....
....
....
....
....
....
....
....
....
....
....
....

Breakfast	Lunch
Dinner	Snacks
--------	--------
Supplements	Medication
-------------	------------

Date ....

Sleep quality and duration ....

Stress levels   1   2   3   4   5   6   7   8   9   10

Time	Systolic	Diastolic	Heart Rate

Exercise and daily activities   Water Intake ☐☐☐☐☐☐☐

....
....
....
....
....
....
....
....
....
....
....
....
....
....
....
....
....

Breakfast	Lunch

Dinner	Snacks

Supplements	Medication

Date ....

Sleep quality and duration ....

Stress levels   1   2   3   4   5   6   7   8   9   10

Time	Systolic	Diastolic	Heart Rate

Exercise and daily activities   Water Intake ☐☐☐☐☐☐☐

....
....
....
....
....
....
....
....
....
....
....
....
....
....
....
....

Breakfast	Lunch

Dinner	Snacks

Supplements	Medication

Date ....

Sleep quality and duration ....

Stress levels 1 2 3 4 5 6 7 8 9 10

Time	Systolic	Diastolic	Heart Rate

Exercise and daily activities   Water Intake ▯▯▯▯▯▯▯

....
....
....
....
....
....

Breakfast	Lunch

....
....
....
....
....

Dinner	Snacks

....
....
....
....
....

Supplements	Medication

Date ....

Sleep quality and duration ....

Stress levels   1   2   3   4   5   6   7   8   9   10

Time	Systolic	Diastolic	Heart Rate

Exercise and daily activities   Water Intake ▢▢▢▢▢▢▢

....
....
....
....
....
....
....
....
....
....
....
....
....
....
....
....
....

Breakfast	Lunch

Dinner	Snacks

Supplements	Medication

Date ....

Sleep quality and duration ....

Stress levels   1   2   3   4   5   6   7   8   9   10

Time	Systolic	Diastolic	Heart Rate

Exercise and daily activities   Water Intake ▯▯▯▯▯▯▯

....
....
....
....
....
....
....
....
....
....
....
....
....
....
....
....

Breakfast	Lunch

Dinner	Snacks

Supplements	Medication

Date ....

Sleep quality and duration ....

Stress levels   1   2   3   4   5   6   7   8   9   10

Time	Systolic	Diastolic	Heart Rate

Exercise and daily activities   Water Intake ☐☐☐☐☐☐☐

....

....

....

Breakfast	Lunch

....

....

....

....

Dinner	Snacks

....

....

....

....

....

Supplements	Medication

....

....

....

....

....

Date ....

Sleep quality and duration ....

Stress levels   1   2   3   4   5   6   7   8   9   10

Time	Systolic	Diastolic	Heart Rate

Exercise and daily activities   Water Intake ▯▯▯▯▯▯▯

....
....
....
....
....
....
....
....
....
....
....
....
....
....
....
....

Breakfast	Lunch

Dinner	Snacks

Supplements	Medication

Date ....

Sleep quality and duration ....

Stress levels   1   2   3   4   5   6   7   8   9   10

Time	Systolic	Diastolic	Heart Rate

Exercise and daily activities   Water Intake ▯▯▯▯▯▯▯

....
....
....
....
....
....
....
....
....
....
....
....
....
....
....
....

Breakfast	Lunch

Dinner	Snacks

Supplements	Medication

Date ....

Sleep quality and duration ....

Stress levels   1   2   3   4   5   6   7   8   9   10

Time	Systolic	Diastolic	Heart Rate

Exercise and daily activities   Water Intake ☐☐☐☐☐☐☐

....
....
....
....
....
....
....
....
....
....
....
....
....
....
....
....

Breakfast	Lunch

Dinner	Snacks

Supplements	Medication

Date ....

Sleep quality and duration ....

Stress levels   1   2   3   4   5   6   7   8   9   10

Time	Systolic	Diastolic	Heart Rate

Exercise and daily activities   Water Intake ☐☐☐☐☐☐☐

....

Breakfast	Lunch

Dinner	Snacks

Supplements	Medication

Date ....

Sleep quality and duration ....

Stress levels   1   2   3   4   5   6   7   8   9   10

Time	Systolic	Diastolic	Heart Rate

Exercise and daily activities   Water Intake ☐☐☐☐☐☐☐

....
....
....
....
....
....
....
....
....
....
....
....
....
....
....

Breakfast	Lunch

Dinner	Snacks

Supplements	Medication

Date ....

Sleep quality and duration ....

Stress levels 1 2 3 4 5 6 7 8 9 10

Time	Systolic	Diastolic	Heart Rate

Exercise and daily activities   Water Intake ▯▯▯▯▯▯▯

....
....
....
....
....
....
....
....
....
....
....
....
....
....
....
....
....

Breakfast	Lunch

Dinner	Snacks

Supplements	Medication

Date ....

Sleep quality and duration ....

Stress levels   1   2   3   4   5   6   7   8   9   10

Time	Systolic	Diastolic	Heart Rate

Exercise and daily activities   Water Intake ☐☐☐☐☐☐☐

....
....
....
....
....
....
....
....
....
....
....
....
....
....
....
....
....

Breakfast	Lunch

Dinner	Snacks

Supplements	Medication

Date ....

Sleep quality and duration ....

Stress levels   1   2   3   4   5   6   7   8   9   10

Time	Systolic	Diastolic	Heart Rate

Exercise and daily activities   Water Intake ☐☐☐☐☐☐☐

....
....
....
....
....
....
....
....
....
....
....
....
....
....
....
....

Breakfast	Lunch

Dinner	Snacks

Supplements	Medication

Date ....

Sleep quality and duration ....

Stress levels   1   2   3   4   5   6   7   8   9   10

Time	Systolic	Diastolic	Heart Rate

Exercise and daily activities   Water Intake ▯▯▯▯▯▯▯

....
....
....
....
....
....

Breakfast	Lunch

....
....
....
....
....

Dinner	Snacks

....
....
....
....
....

Supplements	Medication

Date ....

Sleep quality and duration ....

Stress levels   1   2   3   4   5   6   7   8   9   10

Time	Systolic	Diastolic	Heart Rate

Exercise and daily activities   Water Intake ☐☐☐☐☐☐☐

....
....
....
....
....
....
....
....
....
....
....
....
....
....
....

Breakfast	Lunch
Dinner	Snacks
Supplements	Medication

Date ....

Sleep quality and duration ....

Stress levels   1   2   3   4   5   6   7   8   9   10

Time	Systolic	Diastolic	Heart Rate

Exercise and daily activities   Water Intake ☐☐☐☐☐☐☐

....
....
....
....
....
....
....
....
....
....
....
....
....
....
....
....

Breakfast	Lunch

Dinner	Snacks

Supplements	Medication

Date ....

Sleep quality and duration ....

Stress levels   1   2   3   4   5   6   7   8   9   10

Time	Systolic	Diastolic	Heart Rate

Exercise and daily activities   Water Intake ☐☐☐☐☐☐☐

....
....
....
....
....
....
....
....
....
....
....
....
....
....
....
....

Breakfast	Lunch
Dinner	Snacks
Supplements	Medication

Date ....

Sleep quality and duration ....

Stress levels   1   2   3   4   5   6   7   8   9   10

Time	Systolic	Diastolic	Heart Rate

Exercise and daily activities   Water Intake ▯▯▯▯▯▯▯

....
....
....
....
....
....
....
....
....
....
....
....
....
....
....

Breakfast	Lunch

Dinner	Snacks

Supplements	Medication

Date ....

Sleep quality and duration ....

Stress levels   1   2   3   4   5   6   7   8   9   10

Time	Systolic	Diastolic	Heart Rate

Exercise and daily activities   Water Intake ☐☐☐☐☐☐☐

....
....
....
....
....
....
....
....
....
....
....
....
....
....
....

Breakfast	Lunch

Dinner	Snacks

Supplements	Medication

Date ....

Sleep quality and duration ....

Stress levels   1   2   3   4   5   6   7   8   9
10

Time	Systolic	Diastolic	Heart Rate

Exercise and daily activities   Water Intake ▯▯▯▯▯▯▯

....
....
....
....
....
....
....
....
....
....
....
....
....
....
....
....

Breakfast	Lunch
Dinner	Snacks
Supplements	Medication

Date ....

Sleep quality and duration ....

Stress levels   1   2   3   4   5   6   7   8   9   10

Time	Systolic	Diastolic	Heart Rate

Exercise and daily activities   Water Intake ☐☐☐☐☐☐☐

....
....
....
....
....
....
....
....
....
....
....
....
....
....
....
....

Breakfast	Lunch

Dinner	Snacks

Supplements	Medication

Date ....

Sleep quality and duration ....

Stress levels   1   2   3   4   5   6   7   8   9   10

Time	Systolic	Diastolic	Heart Rate

Exercise and daily activities   Water Intake ▯▯▯▯▯▯▯

....
....
....
....
....
....
....
....
....
....
....
....
....
....
....
....
....

Breakfast	Lunch

Dinner	Snacks

Supplements	Medication

Date ....

Sleep quality and duration ....

Stress levels   1   2   3   4   5   6   7   8   9   10

Time	Systolic	Diastolic	Heart Rate

Exercise and daily activities   Water Intake ☐☐☐☐☐☐☐

....
....
....
....
....
....
....
....
....
....
....
....
....
....
....

Breakfast	Lunch

Dinner	Snacks

Supplements	Medication

Date ....

Sleep quality and duration ....

Stress levels   1   2   3   4   5   6   7   8   9   10

Time	Systolic	Diastolic	Heart Rate

Exercise and daily activities   Water Intake ▯▯▯▯▯▯▯

....
....
....
....
....
....
....
....
....
....
....
....
....
....
....
....

Breakfast	Lunch

Dinner	Snacks

Supplements	Medication

Date ....

Sleep quality and duration ....

Stress levels   1   2   3   4   5   6   7   8   9   10

Time	Systolic	Diastolic	Heart Rate

Exercise and daily activities   Water Intake ▯▯▯▯▯▯▯

....

....

....

Breakfast	Lunch

....

....

....

....

Dinner	Snacks

....

....

....

....

Supplements	Medication

....

....

....

....

Date ....

Sleep quality and duration ....

Stress levels   1   2   3   4   5   6   7   8   9   10

Time	Systolic	Diastolic	Heart Rate

Exercise and daily activities   Water Intake ☐☐☐☐☐☐☐

....
....
....
....
....
....
....
....
....
....
....
....
....
....
....
....
....

Breakfast	Lunch
Dinner	Snacks
Supplements	Medication

Date ....

Sleep quality and duration ....

Stress levels   1   2   3   4   5   6   7   8   9   10

Time	Systolic	Diastolic	Heart Rate

Exercise and daily activities   Water Intake ▯▯▯▯▯▯▯

....
....
....
....
....
....
....
....
....
....
....
....
....
....
....
....

Breakfast	Lunch

Dinner	Snacks

Supplements	Medication

Date ....

Sleep quality and duration ....

Stress levels   1   2   3   4   5   6   7   8   9   10

Time	Systolic	Diastolic	Heart Rate

Exercise and daily activities   Water Intake ☐☐☐☐☐☐☐

....
....
....
....
....
....
....
....
....
....
....
....
....
....
....
....

Breakfast	Lunch
Dinner	**Snacks**
Supplements	Medication

Date ....

Sleep quality and duration ....

Stress levels   1   2   3   4   5   6   7   8   9   10

Time	Systolic	Diastolic	Heart Rate

Exercise and daily activities   Water Intake ☐☐☐☐☐☐☐

....
....
....
....
....
....
....
....
....
....
....
....
....
....
....
....
....

Breakfast	Lunch
Dinner	Snacks
Supplements	Medication

Date ....

Sleep quality and duration ....

Stress levels   1   2   3   4   5   6   7   8   9   10

Time	Systolic	Diastolic	Heart Rate

Exercise and daily activities   Water Intake ☐☐☐☐☐☐☐

....
....
....
....
....
....
....
....
....
....
....
....
....
....
....
....

Breakfast	Lunch

Dinner	Snacks

Supplements	Medication

Date ....

Sleep quality and duration ....

Stress levels   1   2   3   4   5   6   7   8   9   10

Time	Systolic	Diastolic	Heart Rate

Exercise and daily activities   Water Intake ☐☐☐☐☐☐☐

Breakfast	Lunch

Dinner	Snacks

Supplements	Medication

Date ....

Sleep quality and duration ....

Stress levels   1   2   3   4   5   6   7   8   9   10

Time	Systolic	Diastolic	Heart Rate

Exercise and daily activities   Water Intake ☐☐☐☐☐☐☐

....

Breakfast	Lunch

Dinner	Snacks

Supplements	Medication

Date ....

Sleep quality and duration ....

Stress levels   1   2   3   4   5   6   7   8   9   10

Time	Systolic	Diastolic	Heart Rate

Exercise and daily activities   Water Intake ⬜⬜⬜⬜⬜⬜⬜

....

....

Breakfast	Lunch

....

....

....

....

....

Dinner	Snacks

....

....

....

....

Supplements	Medication

....

....

....

....

Date ....

Sleep quality and duration ....

Stress levels   1   2   3   4   5   6   7   8   9   10

Time	Systolic	Diastolic	Heart Rate

Exercise and daily activities   Water Intake ▯▯▯▯▯▯▯

....

....

....

....

....

....

....

....

....

....

....

....

....

....

....

Breakfast	Lunch
Dinner	Snacks
Supplements	Medication

Date ....

Sleep quality and duration ....

Stress levels   1   2   3   4   5   6   7   8   9   10

Time	Systolic	Diastolic	Heart Rate

Exercise and daily activities   Water Intake ☐☐☐☐☐☐☐

....
....
....
....
....
....
....
....
....
....
....
....
....
....
....
....

Breakfast	Lunch
Dinner	Snacks
Supplements	Medication

Date ....

Sleep quality and duration ....

Stress levels   1   2   3   4   5   6   7   8   9   10

Time	Systolic	Diastolic	Heart Rate

Exercise and daily activities   Water Intake ▢▢▢▢▢▢▢

....
....
....
....
....
....
....
....
....
....
....
....
....
....
....
....
....

Breakfast	Lunch

Dinner	Snacks

Supplements	Medication

Date ....

Sleep quality and duration ....

Stress levels   1   2   3   4   5   6   7   8   9   10

Time	Systolic	Diastolic	Heart Rate

Exercise and daily activities   Water Intake ⬜⬜⬜⬜⬜⬜⬜

....

....

Breakfast	Lunch

....

....

....

....

....

Dinner	Snacks

....

....

....

....

Supplements	Medication

....

....

....

....

....

Date ....

Sleep quality and duration ....

Stress levels   1   2   3   4   5   6   7   8   9   10

Time	Systolic	Diastolic	Heart Rate

Exercise and daily activities   Water Intake ☐☐☐☐☐☐☐

....

....

....

....

....

....

....

....

....

....

....

....

....

....

....

Breakfast	Lunch

Dinner	Snacks

Supplements	Medication

Date ....

Sleep quality and duration ....

Stress levels   1   2   3   4   5   6   7   8   9   10

Time	Systolic	Diastolic	Heart Rate

Exercise and daily activities   Water Intake ☐☐☐☐☐☐☐

....
....
....
....
....
....
....
....
....
....
....
....
....
....
....
....
....

Breakfast	Lunch
Dinner	Snacks
Supplements	Medication

Date ....

Sleep quality and duration ....

Stress levels   1   2   3   4   5   6   7   8   9 10

Time	Systolic	Diastolic	Heart Rate

Exercise and daily activities   Water Intake ☐☐☐☐☐☐☐

....

....

....

....

....

....

....

....

....

....

....

....

....

....

....

....

Breakfast	Lunch

Dinner	Snacks

Supplements	Medication

Date ....

Sleep quality and duration ....

Stress levels   1   2   3   4   5   6   7   8   9   10

Time	Systolic	Diastolic	Heart Rate

Exercise and daily activities   Water Intake ☐☐☐☐☐☐☐

....
....
....
....
....
....
....
....
....
....
....
....
....
....
....

Breakfast	Lunch

Dinner	Snacks

Supplements	Medication

Date ....

Sleep quality and duration ....

Stress levels 1 2 3 4 5 6 7 8 9 10

Time	Systolic	Diastolic	Heart Rate

Exercise and daily activities   Water Intake ▯▯▯▯▯▯▯

....
....
....
....
....
....
....
....
....
....
....
....
....
....
....
....
....

Breakfast	Lunch

Dinner	Snacks

Supplements	Medication

Date ....

Sleep quality and duration ....

Stress levels   1   2   3   4   5   6   7   8   9   10

Time	Systolic	Diastolic	Heart Rate

Exercise and daily activities   Water Intake ☐☐☐☐☐☐☐

....
....
....
....
....
....
....
....
....
....
....
....
....
....
....
....

Breakfast	Lunch

Dinner	Snacks

Supplements	Medication

Date ....

Sleep quality and duration ....

Stress levels   1   2   3   4   5   6   7   8   9   10

Time	Systolic	Diastolic	Heart Rate

Exercise and daily activities   Water Intake ▯▯▯▯▯▯▯

....
....
....
....
....
....

Breakfast	Lunch

....
....
....
....

Dinner	Snacks

....
....
....
....
....
....

Supplements	Medication

Date ....

Sleep quality and duration ....

Stress levels   1   2   3   4   5   6   7   8   9   10

Time	Systolic	Diastolic	Heart Rate

Exercise and daily activities   Water Intake ☐☐☐☐☐☐☐

....
....
....
....
....
....
....
....
....
....
....
....
....
....
....
....
....

Breakfast	Lunch

Dinner	Snacks

Supplements	Medication

Date ....

Sleep quality and duration ....

Stress levels   1   2   3   4   5   6   7   8   9   10

Time	Systolic	Diastolic	Heart Rate

Exercise and daily activities   Water Intake ☐☐☐☐☐☐☐

....
....
....
....
....
....
....
....
....
....
....
....
....
....
....
....

Breakfast	Lunch

Dinner	Snacks

Supplements	Medication

Date ....

Sleep quality and duration ....

Stress levels 1 2 3 4 5 6 7 8 9 10

Time	Systolic	Diastolic	Heart Rate

Exercise and daily activities   Water Intake ☐☐☐☐☐☐☐

....
....
....
....
....
....
....
....
....
....
....
....
....
....
....
....

Breakfast	Lunch

Dinner	Snacks

Supplements	Medication

Date ....

Sleep quality and duration ....

Stress levels 1 2 3 4 5 6 7 8 9 10

Time	Systolic	Diastolic	Heart Rate

Exercise and daily activities   Water Intake ☐☐☐☐☐☐

....
....
....
....
....
....
....
....
....
....
....
....
....
....
....
....
....

Breakfast	Lunch

Dinner	Snacks

Supplements	Medication

Date ....

Sleep quality and duration ....

Stress levels   1   2   3   4   5   6   7   8   9   10

Time	Systolic	Diastolic	Heart Rate

Exercise and daily activities   Water Intake ☐☐☐☐☐☐☐

....
....
....
....
....
....
....
....
....
....
....
....
....
....
....
....

Breakfast	Lunch

Dinner	Snacks

Supplements	Medication

Date ....

Sleep quality and duration ....

Stress levels   1   2   3   4   5   6   7   8   9   10

Time	Systolic	Diastolic	Heart Rate

Exercise and daily activities   Water Intake ☐☐☐☐☐☐☐

....
....
....
....
....
....
....
....
....
....
....
....
....
....
....
....
....

Breakfast	Lunch

Dinner	Snacks

Supplements	Medication

Date ....

Sleep quality and duration ....

Stress levels   1   2   3   4   5   6   7   8   9   10

Time	Systolic	Diastolic	Heart Rate

Exercise and daily activities   Water Intake ▯▯▯▯▯▯▯

....
....
....
....
....
....
....
....
....
....
....
....
....
....
....
....

Breakfast	Lunch

Dinner	Snacks

Supplements	Medication

Date ....

Sleep quality and duration ....

Stress levels   1   2   3   4   5   6   7   8   9   10

Time	Systolic	Diastolic	Heart Rate

Exercise and daily activities   Water Intake ☐☐☐☐☐☐☐

....

....

....

Breakfast	Lunch

....

....

....

....

....

Dinner	Snacks

....

....

....

....

....

Supplements	Medication

....

....

....

....

....

Date ....

Sleep quality and duration ....

Stress levels   1   2   3   4   5   6   7   8   9   10

Time	Systolic	Diastolic	Heart Rate

Exercise and daily activities   Water Intake ☐☐☐☐☐☐☐

....
....
....
....
....
....
....
....
....
....
....
....
....
....
....
....
....

Breakfast	Lunch

Dinner	Snacks

Supplements	Medication

Date ....

Sleep quality and duration ....

Stress levels   1   2   3   4   5   6   7   8   9   10

Time	Systolic	Diastolic	Heart Rate

Exercise and daily activities   Water Intake ☐☐☐☐☐☐☐

....
....
....
....
....
....
....
....
....
....
....
....
....
....
....
....
....

Breakfast	Lunch

Dinner	Snacks

Supplements	Medication

Date ....

Sleep quality and duration ....

Stress levels   1   2   3   4   5   6   7   8   9   10

Time	Systolic	Diastolic	Heart Rate

Exercise and daily activities   Water Intake ▯▯▯▯▯▯▯

....
....
....
....
....
....
....
....
....
....
....
....
....
....
....
....

Breakfast	Lunch

Dinner	Snacks

Supplements	Medication

Date ....

Sleep quality and duration ....

Stress levels 1 2 3 4 5 6 7 8 9
10

Time	Systolic	Diastolic	Heart Rate

Exercise and daily activities   Water Intake ☐☐☐☐☐☐

....
....
....
....
....
....
....
....
....
....
....
....
....
....
....
....

Breakfast	Lunch
Dinner	Snacks
Supplements	Medication

Date ....

Sleep quality and duration ....

Stress levels   1   2   3   4   5   6   7   8   9   10

Time	Systolic	Diastolic	Heart Rate

Exercise and daily activities   Water Intake ▯▯▯▯▯▯▯

....
....
....
....
....
....
....
....
....
....
....
....
....
....
....
....

Breakfast	Lunch

Dinner	Snacks

Supplements	Medication

Date ....

Sleep quality and duration ....

Stress levels   1   2   3   4   5   6   7   8   9   10

Time	Systolic	Diastolic	Heart Rate

Exercise and daily activities   Water Intake ▢▢▢▢▢▢▢

....

....

....

....

....

....

....

....

....

....

....

....

....

....

....

....

Breakfast	Lunch

Dinner	Snacks

Supplements	Medication

Date ....

Sleep quality and duration ....

Stress levels   1   2   3   4   5   6   7   8   9   10

Time	Systolic	Diastolic	Heart Rate

Exercise and daily activities   Water Intake ▢▢▢▢▢▢▢

....
....
....
....
....
....
....
....
....
....
....
....
....
....
....
....

Breakfast	Lunch
Dinner	Snacks
Supplements	Medication

Date ....

Sleep quality and duration ....

Stress levels   1   2   3   4   5   6   7   8   9   10

Time	Systolic	Diastolic	Heart Rate

Exercise and daily activities   Water Intake ▯▯▯▯▯▯

....
....
....
....
....
....
....
....
....
....
....
....
....
....
....
....

Breakfast	Lunch

Dinner	Snacks

Supplements	Medication

Date ....

Sleep quality and duration ....

Stress levels 1 2 3 4 5 6 7 8 9 10

Time	Systolic	Diastolic	Heart Rate

Exercise and daily activities   Water Intake ☐☐☐☐☐☐☐

....

....

....

Breakfast	Lunch

....

....

....

....

Dinner	Snacks

....

....

....

....

Supplements	Medication

....

....

....

....

....

Thank you

We hope you enjoyed our book
As a small family company,
your feedback is very important to us.
Please let us know how you like our book at :
PROMOBILEAMZ@GMAIL.COM

Doctor B. Telep

www.ingramcontent.com/pod-product-compliance
Lightning Source LLC
LaVergne TN
LVHW011729060526
838200LV00051B/3097